Vagus Nerve: Beginner's Guide

How to Activate the Natural Healing Power of Your Body with Exercises to Overcome Anxiety, Depression, Trauma, Inflammation, Brain Fog, and Improve Your Life.

Amy Kingswood

© **Copyright 2021 - All rights reserved.**

The content contained within this book may not be reproduced, duplicated or transmitted without direct written permission from the author or the publisher.

Under no circumstances will any blame or legal responsibility be held against the publisher, or author, for any damages, reparation, or monetary loss due to the information contained within this book, either directly or indirectly.

Legal Notice:

This book is copyright protected. It is only for personal use. You cannot amend, distribute, sell, use, quote or paraphrase any part, or the content within this book, without the consent of the author or publisher.

Disclaimer Notice:

Please note the information contained within this document is for educational and entertainment purposes only. All effort has been executed to present accurate, up to date, reliable, complete information. No warranties of any kind are declared or implied. Readers acknowledge that the author is not engaged in the rendering of legal, financial, medical or professional advice. The content within this book has been derived from various sources. Please consult a licensed professional before attempting any techniques outlined in this book.

By reading this document, the reader agrees that under no circumstances is the author responsible for any losses, direct or indirect, that are incurred as a result of the use of the information contained within this document, including, but not limited to, errors, omissions, or inaccuracies.

Table of Contents

Introduction

Chapter One: Anatomy of the Vagus Nerve and its Relation to Exercise

Chapter Two: Vagus Nerve and Health Status

Chapter Three: Injury to the Vagus nerve

Chapter Four: Polyvagal Theory

Conclusion

Introduction

The vagus nerve is called "wandering nerve" in Latin. It is one of the most crucial cranial nerves in the body; it's considered the longest cranial nerve, running between the brain and the gastrointestinal tract. While it is paired, it is often viewed as a singular nerve.

The vagus nerve performs diverse bodily functions, from parasympathetic functions to the motor, sensory, and even special sensory. As such, it generally affects the overall wellness of the human body. It participates in homeostasis, which is the regulation of the body system.

It has an extensive distribution around the body, from the face and neck to the thorax, and the more significant part of the abdomen (gastrointestinal tract). Understanding how extensive the vagus nerve is in its distribution and the parts of the body it is supplying will give us a comprehensive understanding of how to stimulate the vagus nerve single-handedly and naturally to get results.

Many people are not familiar with the vagus nerve or don't even know about its presence or how it functions, so it will be difficult for us to see the power we have with its presence in the body and what happens when it gets damaged or injured.

We must understand how certain things in our bodies work for us to live quality lives. Understanding the vagus nerve, its distribution, stimulation, and the power attached to it will bring a massive revolution to our lives. Sometimes when we become goal-driven and highly focused, we neglect our health and fall into stress which affects our mind from functioning properly, eventually reducing our productivity level. Needless to say, our level of productivity is directly connected with our mind's stability and mental soundness.

If you are not in a good state of mind, you cannot get anything done, and this will hamper you from reaching your overall life goals because you are not in touch with yourself and lack alignment between your body, soul, and spirit.

It becomes crucial you understand natural strategies you can bank on anytime to relieve yourself of the built-up stress that will result in anxiety, depression, inflammation, trauma, brain fog, or any combination of these.

Most times, we are overwhelmed and stressed out because we do not sit and identify our stressors. Also, we do not recognize when we have reached our limits and need to retreat, rest and revitalize until frustration sets in and we can no longer cope with the situations around us.

Every human carries a natural super-power that makes natural healing possible due to the power of the mind. If you can get your mind in order, then you can achieve a vast level of results.

Inhibitors like anxiety, depression, confusion, brain fog, can set in due to the stress around us, and they can be better handled naturally through the super-power that comes through the vagus nerve.

The vagus nerve is an interface between the brain and the body; when stimulated, it has several health benefits. It reduces the heartbeat, circulation, digestion, and circulation by triggering the release of a neurotransmitter called "acetylcholine" in our nervous system.

When these are regulated, these activities are reduced, and the body naturally regains its health. The functions the vagus nerve performs in restoring our health after trauma and fight/flight actions cannot be overemphasized. Everyone can tap into this superpower of the vagus nerve to build confidence and a sound mind, which can help you normalize these activities over a long period once you master these vagus nerve stimulation processes.

Vagus nerve dysfunction can occur due to different things like infection, injury to the vagus nerve, damage to the nerve due to brain injury, damage to the nerve that may arise during the surgery, for example, stomach surgery.

Stephen Porges discovered polyvagal theory, and he explained three stages of responses: immobilization, mobilization, and social engagement. Immobilization is the stage where we are caught up with a parasympathetic phase, which the vagus nerve is participatory in, where an individual goes numb or even shuts down when faced with danger or fearful events around him.

Mobilization is the stage of fight or flight when we are swung into motion when faced with danger or scary situations. This happens in a bid for us to either take action to confront the enemy by defending ourselves or run for our dear lives. This occurs when the adrenaline has been released.

The polyvagal theory deals with our social interactions, connections, communications, and disconnections with our environment. Facial and vocalization are very crucial in our social harmony and determines our connection or disconnection with others.

A traumatized individual may not have the flight or fight signals because of the vegeatative state he or she finds his or herself in overtime and, as such, may need help to adjust to the environment and learn between different signals to feel safe and secure, or know when to take actions.

The significance of the vagus nerve cannot be overemphasized. We must treat it with cautiousness because damage to the vagus nerve will result in the dysfunction or imbalance of the general body system and impair the general body functioning.

When you understand these things and how to leverage these features of the vagus nerve, you will experience an improvement in every area of your life, including your mental health, and your mental health will invariably affect your productivity.

Research has shown that people do different things subconsciously that connect with the vagus nerve and help them recover from depression unknowingly. Laughter, singing, intermittent fasting, dancing are some of these activities. These exercises activate our vagus nerves and give us natural healing from inhibitions like depression.

Others include increased intake of fibers, gum chewing, 4:8 breathing exercises, and sleeping on the right-hand side.

Knowing the vagus nerve and the supernatural healing that comes with its stimulation will help us be more intentional about the activities we engage in and help us stay mentally healthy. We can leverage this knowledge to get our healing anytime, any day.

This book contains valuable insights that will change your perspectives about exercise and show you the natural superpower you carry in your body that can bring healing to your soul without needing to visit hospitals or take drugs. Enjoy the read!

Chapter One: Anatomy of the Vagus Nerve and its Relation to Exercise

The vagus nerve is essential to the body. It is the tenth of the twelve cranial nerves and originated from the base of the brain. It is known as the wandering nerve because of the multiple branches it sends out of the brain to the whole body.

Even though it is often seen as a singular nerve and not paired, the vagus nerve is complex. It runs through the face to the gastrointestinal organs and the internal organs. The vagus nerve is a mixed nerve which is considered the parasympathetic nerve. It has two sensory ganglia that transmit sensory information and function in the regulation of the body system.

It has an 80% afferent distribution and 20% efferent distribution. The vagus nerve distributes its branches extensively in the body with two ganglia. The superior ganglion, which is also called jugular ganglion, of the vagus nerve supplies the major part of the ear. The concha of the auricle, the posterior-inferior part of the tympanic membrane and some other areas of the ear through its branch called an auricular nerve.

The inferior ganglion, also known as lower ganglion, is located just below the superior ganglion has two branches. They are the pharyngeal nerve and the superior laryngeal nerve.

The recurrent laryngeal nerve has its branch from the vagus at the lower part of the neck and upper part of the thorax to supply the muscles of the larynx (the voice box). The vagus nerve also sends out the cardiac, esophageal, and pulmonary branches. The vagus nerve supplies the larger part of the digestive tract in the abdomen and internal organs.

The vagus nerve also conveys the sensory signals from the body's internal organs to the brain, which helps the brain to monitor the internal organs' actions.

The vagus nerve helps to give the primary control for the parasympathetic part of the nervous system of the body. The rest-and-digest system counterbalances the fight-or-flight response of the sympathetic part of the nervous system.

When the body is not being subjected to stress or pressure, the vagus nerve sends off information that slows down the heart and breathing rates and increases the action of the digestive system. But when the body is under stress, the vagus nerve shifts the control to the sympathetic system, which gives the opposite effect.

The vagus was generally believed to be an efferent nerve and also the counterpoint of the sympathetic nervous system. The majority of these organs receive parasympathetic efferents via the vagus nerve and sympathetic efferents also via the splanchnic nerves.

The vagal afferent nerves aid the regulation of the HPA (hypothalamus-pituitary-adrenal) axis which helps to control the adaptive responses of humans to stressors around them.

Different stressors affect different people. Stress can occur as a result of environmental stressors which may include changes in weather conditions, noise, heat, or chemical substances. You must study yourself to know whether your stressors are environmentally related.

These stressors activate corticotropin-releasing factor (CRF), which is from the hypothalamus, and in return, release adrenocorticotropic hormone from the pituitary gland. It travels into the blood and causes the release of cortisol hormone, the stress hormone.

Humans respond to stressors differently; the response could be pain, anxiety, depression, or inflammation, depending on the individual body system, as a result of the release of the stress hormones in the body.

High levels of adrenocorticotropic hormone cause depression, anxiety, nervous conditions, anorexia nervosa, insomnia, and even inflammatory conditions.

These stress hormones are adrenaline, cortisol, and norepinephrine. These stress hormones cause an increase in the heart rate and high blood pressure, which must be reduced after the event lest it results in death, which is what the vagus nerve corrects.

The CRF release stimulates adrenocorticotropic hormone (ACTH) secretion from the pituitary gland. This stimulation results in the release of cortisol from the adrenal glands. Cortisol is one of the major stress hormones, as said earlier, and it affects several organs in the body, including the brain, bones, muscles, and also body fat.

These hormones are released moderately into the body in the morning when you wake up from sleep. These releases of hormones help to regulate your heartbeat and blood pressure and strengthen your mood for the day ahead.

Collectively, the sympathetic nervous systems and the parasympathetic nervous system are responsible for the regulation of body functions which helps to improve the quality of life.

Understanding the anatomy of the vagus nerves, their extensive distribution, and the stimulation of the various branches and their effects will help us to understand how effectively we can maximize the natural healing power it supplies.

Chapter Two: Vagus Nerve and Health Status

The vagus nerve is involved in the general wellness of the body. It participates in the regulation of some of the most important physiological functions in the body, and your overall health depends on the health of this nerve.

The vagus nerve carries most of the information from the gut, esophagus, larynx, and abdomen, as well as other internal organs to the brain for regulation. The vagusstoff substance released by the stimulation of the vagus nerve is responsible for increasing our vagal tone to help us relax faster when the body is under stress.

Vagal tone is the activity of the vagus nerve, and the rate of the vagal tone determines how fast or slow the body relaxes after a stressful event or adrenaline-fueled fight-or-flight response.

The vagal tone also determines the health of an individual as it determines the heart rate, the pressure of the blood, digestions, and the risk of getting cardiovascular diseases.

A low vagal tone means the body will be slow to relax and the heartbeat remains high with high blood pressure, anxiety disorder, trauma, and affects general functioning of the body.

A high vagal tone means the body will relax fast after stress or a fight or flight incidence; it helps to reduce the risk of stroke, cardiac arrest, and high blood pressure. It also aids blood sugar regulation and digestion, and it also helps to prevent inflammatory conditions like lupus, arthritis, and autoimmune typhoid conditions.

There are several ways one can stimulate the vagus nerve to increase the vagal tone for the homeostatic functioning of the body. One of them is by engaging in exercises, as mentioned earlier. The most important exercises are ones that involve controlled breathing (breathing more slowly) or engage in relaxation techniques. These include singing, dancing, yoga, and meditation.

So many people die of different diseases that could have been prevented or stopped by just exercises, but lack of knowledge of how to get natural healing through exercises or normal activity result in their deaths.

Obesity has been recorded to be one of the deadliest diseases. It is a result of the body fat or cholesterol deposits in the body which results in high blood pressure, increased heart rate, fatigue, and others.

If an obese individual could engage in some of these activities to stimulate the vagus nerve and burn more fat, then his or her blood pressure will be normalized, which can help the patient reduce the tendency of having cardiovascular diseases or cardiac arrest from the high blood pressure.

Also, when you learn to engage in exercises more often, you will have the power to stop the tendency to fall into depression or anxiety as a result of stress. Sometimes work can be overwhelming, and we keep managing the stress poorly until we break down.

It can be frustrating, but exercises like jogging, meditation can help you clear your mind, unwind, and give you a healthy mind, empowering you to refocus to hit your goals. This, in turn, improves your life by helping you toward the goal of a happy life. But with depression, anxiety, and brain fog, everything becomes frustrating and annoying.

I once heard about a case of a woman who visited the hospital to complain of a headache now and then; the doctor prescribed drugs for her, but she kept going back to complain about the same headache. The doctor kept wondering if she was taking her drugs as prescribed; she nodded in affirmation.

Then, the doctor took a step further to know if there was any stress she was under. The woman opened up about her marriage, and the doctor soon realized that the woman had been struggling with her marriage, and it was this that was stressing her out, leading to mental stress and brain fog.

She requested that the woman go back and resolve the issue immediately and return as no matter the drug prescribed for her, she wouldn't recover from the headache until she deals with the stressor. She agreed and went back home.

A few days later she came back happy but the headache persisted. Then, the doctor took her through a few exercises, like deep breathing, that involve focusing on the exercise rather than the pain and also recommended early morning jogging and yoga. A week later, she was back to normal and regained her happy mood.

Stress is a very dangerous thing and can endanger life if care is not taken; you must know when you have reached your limit and need to take a break to unwind and clear your mind so as to prevent deep depression, anxiety, and occasional anger.

There are different kinds of stressors that can stress an individual; we have different bodily designs and systems, and as such, we may react to things differently. It is essential everyone understands themselves and knows what stresses them if they want to live healthy lives and avoid constantly being stressed, anxious, or depressed.

Oftentimes, depression and anxiety come as a result of prolonged stress in the body, and when you don't know what you have exposed yourself to that resulted in stress, you may keep exposing yourself to it without knowing, and this may lead to different illnesses in your body.

Stressors can be chemical, physical, or biological agents. They can also be environmental conditions, events, and even external stimuli. Stress results in mental, physical, and chemical responses in the body and may lead to a decrease in mental functioning and productivity.

An individual may be stressed as a result of too many demands from his or her job while another person can be stressed as a result of being in a crowd or too much noise around them. This can depend on your wiring and body system. However, the most important thing is that the presence of the vagus nerve in the body can lead one to heal naturally through its own stimulation.

Someone may be stressed because of relationship or marital issues, too much negative attention from family, friends, or children. It may even be a combination of these that result in stress. All these may result in depression and anxiety and reduce productivity.

The continuous stimulation of the vagus nerve helps to outgrow these stressors by suppressing their effects on your body; you can, metaphorically, grow a thick skin to those things that normally stress you when you have a high vagal tone. This is why you must incorporate breathing exercises and relaxation techniques into your activities often, especially if you are the type that responds easily to stressors around you.

My stressors are crowds and noise; I don't like these two. I get tired and drained when I have to be exposed to too much constant noise or large crowds. However, I saw the need to deal with these stressors, and I decided that I was going to work and be successful at managing them. I began to prepare my mind by starting to practice meditation exercises and deep breathing, which are explained in the next chapter.

I saw remarkable changes in my life.

Today, I can deal with crowds, and no amount of noise can stress me out. I thrive more now because of the mental strength having a high vagal tone has given me.

Exercises That Stimulate The Vagus Nerve

The vagus is the most crucial among the cranial nerves because the major assignment is the aid communication between the brain, ear, and internal organs, which means the vagus nerve tells the brain whatever is going on in the body it is innervating.

For effectiveness in our exercises and other relaxation techniques, we must understand how exercises affect the vagus nerve to help stimulate it to improve our general body wellness. It means if there is any dysfunction or disorder in the vagus nerve, the entire body will malfunction.

During exercises, the vagus nerve is stimulated, and its stimulation leads to the release of the substance called the vagustoff, which, in turn, helps to counterbalance the effect of the adrenaline in the body.

We can leverage the vagus nerve to overcome depression, anxiety disorder, trauma, and also improve the quality of lives through exercises, relaxation techniques, unwinding, singing, dancing, and even meditation. All these exercises are essential and must be practiced until one of them becomes your lifestyle.

No doubt, exercises are good for the body, especially helping it overcome brain fog, which is mental stress and normally occurs as a result of piled-up stress in the body. When an individual refuses to get rid of stress over a long time, like weeks or months, it may lead to chronic fatigue, which eventually results in brain fog.

Also, we must understand that excess activation of this nerve in the body is detrimental to human health, especially women's health. The overactivation mostly results in emotional stress (when your emotions are imbalanced, leading to unnecessary eruptions of anger or rage-like emotions). This is a result of the parasympathetic nervous system overcompensating for the work of the sympathetic nervous system.

When the vagus nerve is overstimulated, it may also result in a low blood supply to the cerebral. This happens as a result of the drop in cardiac output, which occurs when the vagusstoff is stimulated to reverse the work of the adrenaline in the body to reduce the blood pressure and flow. This may pose serious danger to human health by causing brain problems due to a shortage of supply of nutrients to the brain through the blood supply.

How Do Exercises Increase the Vagal Tone?

Vagal tone, as explained earlier, is the activity of the vagus nerve that is responsible for the body's physiological functions. The most important thing is to be consistent with these exercises until it becomes habitual and is part of your daily routine. You stand a chance of living longer when you get used to engaging in exercises.

Vagus nerve stimulation can be defined as any form of technique that helps to stimulate the vagus nerve for an increased vagal tone and decreased heart rate variations. It can be stimulated through different breathing and relaxation techniques.

Chapter Three: Injury to the Vagus Nerve

We have established the fact that the vagus nerve is responsible for the general wellness of the entire body as a result of its stimulation. The reason why many people dwell so long in depression and have prolonged anxiety is that they have not understood the leverage the stimulation of the vagus nerve has for them to experience natural healing in their mood and mind.

Anxiety, worry, depression, brain fog, obesity, and chronic inflammation can be as a result of damage to the vagus nerve, or its improper functioning of the vagus nerve, in the body as well as neurotransmitter imbalances. When you can successfully get this nerve to function well, it means you have reversed all these automatically.

There are other symptoms of vagus nerve we should pay attention to which include nutrient deficiency most importantly vitamin B, irregular insulin level, arrhythmias, different kinds of motion sickness, gastrointestinal problems, fatigue, poor memory, lack of focus, digestion problems, constipation, liver dysfunction, difficulty swallowing food and saliva, and consistent fainting.

Sometimes when you stand too long outside in the sun, you may feel faint repeatedly, and it may seem like there is a big problem. However, the issue sometimes is with the vagus nerve; when there is a dysfunction or pressure on the vagus nerve and there is an insufficient supply of oxygen to the brain, then you will shut down.

The truth is that you can get your vagus nerve stimulated without any external assistance, you only need the knowledge of it to do it yourself.

There was a time I was experiencing a multitude of overlapping challenges in my life, and as a result of this, I fell into depression and became nervous and scared of things that haven't even happened to me. I stayed for years in this depression; I became withdrawn from people until I learned to stimulate my vagus nerve through singing and dancing. When that happened, I began to regain my mind, then I was healed naturally from depression and anxiety.

Damage to the vagus nerve can also result in extreme outcomes. Traumatic brain injury is also known as a silent epidemic disease. It can occur as a result of damage to the vagus nerve or pressure on the nerve. People with traumatic brain injury battle decreased blood pressure, hypoperfusion, edema, inflammations, and a decrease in the level of oxygen that is being supplied to the brain, which is as a result of the dysfunction in the branches of the vagus nerves carrying information to the brain.

From several pieces of research, it was found out that the vagus nerve stimulation will bring about healing in traumatic brain injuries. Vagus nerve stimulation has been done through other means aside from a natural way of stimulating the vagus nerve in the hospital and patients have recovered.

Anyone suffering from trauma can leverage the natural healing that comes through the stimulation of the vagus nerve to get this healing without much force.

Different people have reported that stimulating their vagus nerve has led to an enhancement in their mood; they feel happier and their outlook is brighter. There was also increased memory and recall as well as an ability to connect more with their environment, understand things deeper, and a distinct improvement in their cognition. Their sleepiness in the daytime decreased and appetite for food normalized. This has helped them in their general well-being.

Vagus nerve dysfunction has also been connected to the hoarseness of voice, difficulty in breathing, difficulty in swallowing, tightness in the throat and chest. This dysfunction may occur as a result of damage or pressure on the vagus nerve.

Vagus nerve can get damaged as a result of an infection or may be affected by surgery to the stomach or injury to the nerve itself. Most of the recommendations presented for these cases, especially the hoarseness of the voice, are for vagus nerve stimulation, which results in relaxation and healing.

One of the branches of the vagus nerve, the laryngeal nerve, innervates the larynx, which is the voice box. This means that any injury to either the branch or the parent nerve will automatically affect the area being supplied. When you notice cracking in your voice, you can stimulate your vagus nerve till you regain your voice.

One thing about the vagus nerve injury is that, if detected early, it is possible to prevent patients from having certain complications that come with its damage, which may have long-term complications.

How To Treat the Vagus Nerve Injury

Examples of exercises that stimulate the vagus nerve include the following.

Deep Breathing

This involves slow movement of the belly; this helps you to move your focus from the pain and stress you are experiencing to the breathing exercises, Because, alternatively, once you focus on your pain and decide to hold your breath, it results in pain and stiffness thereby increasing the fight/flight response and the cardiac output.

Breathing Exercise

This involves breathing in for your diaphragm to enlarge, then counting from one to five, then releasing your breath through the mouth (which you should make into a small whole). This is when you are in fight/flight mode and need to calm down. You can have up to ten to fourteen breaths, and releasing your breath through the mouth and not through the nose makes it more of a conscious process and you tend to focus on the rhythmic of the breathing instead of the pain thereby making it effective.

This activates the work of the parasympathetic system and suppresses the sympathetic system activities, thereby reducing cardiac output and heart rate variations, all as a result of the stimulation of the vagus nerve.

Deep breathing exercise which is breathing from the belly may be very painful but with endurance principle, you focus on your breath and forget about the pain to reduce the stress and pain that comes as a result of the flight/fight response.

Your muscles are relaxed as a result of the switching to the parasympathetic system leading to the reduction in anxiety and worry; there is an increase in the oxygen supply to the body cells which helps to produce an endorphin hormone which is normally called "feel-good" hormone in the body.

The Breathing Technique

1. Breathe in slowly and think of having 6-7 breaths in a minute

2. Breathe in from your belly (deeply), enlarge your abdomen, and expand your rib cage as you breathe in.

3. Breathe out more than you breathe in; exhalation activates relaxation due to the vagusstoff production and the stress; pain and pressure will drop off.

More on Breathing Techniques

Over the years, it has been established that there is definitely a connection between longer exhalation and relaxation via the vagus nerve. The vagus nerve calms down the body. This is why another breathing technique, the 4:8 breathing technique, works like magic in relieving stress, relaxing the body, strengthening your mind, and even giving you gut feelings. The vagus nerve is very powerful.

I became fatigued one evening, and I was too tired to even consider jogging as an option to relieve the stress. I had spoken to a friend, who was a therapist, a few months before, and they had told me about 4:8 breathing technique. So, I resorted to engaging in it. Surprisingly, after the five rounds of 4:8 breathing techniques, I had to lay down and rest and that was all, I slept like never before because I felt so relaxed. So, how does it work?

4:8 breathing technique involves exhaling twice as much as you inhale. This means that if you inhale once, you exhale back twice. When you inhale four times and exhale eight times non-stop; that's weird right? And seemingly difficult. But it works like a charm.

This technique works like meditation. It gets your mind focused as you unwind during the exhalation. But the only way you can get the best out of it is to set a goal for it before starting; know how many inhalations and exhalations you are going for before even starting at all to avoid distraction and interruptions in between. When you learn to do this often, your vagal tone will increase, and this will bring you into a healthy and stable mental state. Fatigue, stress, brain fog, depression, and trauma may set in but definitely won't last long in your body.

Singing and Humming

The vagus nerve has branches that supply or innervate the larynx (the voice box); when singing and humming, it is stimulated for relaxation and a clear mind. This is why you are just happy and free of worries and anxieties, especially when you listen to your favorite song from your playlist and sing with the artist.

When you incorporate singing or humming into your daily activities you will observe that you are free from every form of stress and always happy because it increases your vagal tone.

Meditation

Meditation is very powerful when it comes to calming down the body and bringing the body into relaxation mode because it stimulates the vagus nerve and sends a signal to the brain that there is no need to fight or take flight.

Meditation works by bringing your mind to a calm state and renewing your focus; when you learn to meditate often, you will be far from anxiety and unnecessary worry by increasing your vagal tone for better mental and physical functioning.

Wim Hof Relaxation Method

This technique was named after the person who discovered it, Wim Hof. He discovered that exposure to cold has a great effect on your vagus nerve and has the power to bring the body to a relaxed state. Wim Hof explained that exposure to cold reduces stress, pains, energizes, and even relieves symptoms of arthritis and other diseases associated with fight/flight response in the body.

Wim Hof also revealed that this method helps to renew focus, bring the mind into a stable state for productivity, and also stabilizes every other area of your life. This method is often practiced by professional athletes and other successful people who engage in high levels of mental activities and need their mind to be stable as often as possible.

There have been several testimonies about the Wim Hof Method; those who were consistent with cold baths or showers and were healed from arthritis, brain fog, and other ailments. The Wim Hof Method is a great and reliable method indeed.

Intermittent Fasting

Fasting has a way of bringing your body to rest and relaxation mode by aiding your digestion. Also, when you take a break from taking snacks and junks, your body can digest the food speedily, thereby stimulating the vagus nerve and helping in improving your health and the quality of your life.

Laughter

This affects the branches of the vagus nerve sent to the facial muscles and when an individual laughs, these nerves are stimulated. Laughter also helps to release different neurotransmitters in the body that aids the relaxation of the body by helping to send signals to the brain that there is no fight/flight event going on, and as such, the body should relax.

This is why it is generally believed that laughter improves your health and even makes you look younger due to an increased vagal tone in the body.

Body Massage

Massages also help to increase the vagal tone which helps the brain to unwind, helps to relieve stress and even heal depression because there are releases of lymphatics into the body as well, which help fight toxins.

These exercises are great and help to increase the vagal tone for homeostasis to take place. It helps you get better sleep, supplies you with energy, regulates blood flow and pressure and gives you high mental strength thereby improving the quality of your life.

There are several things the vagus nerve does in the body and has great connections with the state of our health. We must avoid damage to the vagus nerve at all costs to avoid malfunction in the body.

Meditating on Gratitude and Kindness

Anything that involves meditation is very powerful, but when it involves gratitude, then it is more powerful. Sometimes we are caught up with different things in our mind and we forget the little successes, the little opportunities coming our way, or how far we have gone in life, then we enter depression; we become anxious because we lose touch with ourselves and the reality of things around us.

Gratitude is the recognition of things that have happened to us and through us and we are grateful for it; the truth is many of us may not be where we desire to be yet but we must understand that we are not where we used to be and be sincerely grateful for it.

Meditation on gratitude and kindness of God helps to stimulate the vagus nerve, which, in turn, helps us unwind, clear our mind and reset our focus. This helps us to step out of depression and anxiety, and we get a renewed mind to keep moving.

Meditation is an exercise, and although it is not an easy one (getting your mind to stay focused and picking up what to think and meditate on take practice), when we begin to give ourselves to this, we will surely become a changed person and our lives will improve greatly.

Probiotics and Prebiotics

The vagus nerve is the nerve that aids the communication between the gut and the brain. The gut has microbiota that keeps it healthy and our general wellness is determined by our gut health as well.

The gut's microbiota has a remarkable influence on the vagus nerve and, as such, we must ensure that these gut microbiota must be kept intact. Lactobacillus rhamnosus and Bifidobacterium longum have been linked to the reduction of depression and anxiety; these two are powerful prebiotic strains.

Other probiotic strains have been established through research to also have an effect on the vagus nerve; they stimulate it to relieve stress in animals and probably in humans as well.

Seafood

There are some seafood that have been linked to vagus nerve stimulation. These include omega-3 fatty acids of EPA and DHA, which are mostly found in fish. These are very essential in the body as they stimulate the vagus nerve and help to relieve stress, heal anxiety, and depression and also improve the quality of life generally.

Healthy Social Connection

Having healthy relationships in your life has a great effect on your vagus nerve. The love, compassion, and happiness that comes from genuine relationships help to modulate your mood and prevent you from entering depression and anxiety even when certain situations warrant it.

Ensure you avoid negative people by all means if you want to improve your life. Negative people suppress your vagus nerve through their negative words, which will keep you in a bad mood because you will be mentally and emotionally stressed by them.

Sunlight

The sunlight has a very important function it performs in the body. One of the functions of sunlight is to stimulate the melanocyte stimulating hormone (MSH) which has a great impact on the vagus nerve. It helps to stimulate the vagus nerve directly.

Ultraviolet rays help to multiply the number of Melanocyte stimulating hormone receptors in the body thereby increasing the tendencies at which it binds.

Sleep Patterns and Vagus Nerve Stimulation

From research, it was found out that sleeping on the back is one of the things that decreases the vagus nerve stimulation while sleeping on the right-hand side helps to stimulate it, thereby causing a decrease in the heartbeat, blood flow, and cardiac output.

Reducing Gluten Consumption and Vagus Nerve Stimulation

Gluten has been recognized as one of the substances that reduce the vagus nerve's normal functioning. Glutens hinder the stimulation of the vagus nerve and as such must be avoided in our foods.

Foods that contain gluten include: breads, pastas, baked foods, stouts (which contain barley), biscuits, and certain fries. Research the foods that are among your favorites, and check their contents before consumption. This will help us improve health and the quality of life.

Increasing Fiber Intake

Fibers are good digestive materials and have been known over the decades for this important function they perform in the body. Fibers aid digestion because of their production of the hormone known as the GLP-1 hormone, which stimulates the vagus nerve, thereby resulting in smooth digestion in the body.

Fibers also help to reduce appetite and make one feel full with just a little food intake; this helps to reduce the risk of obesity and high blood pressure that can invariably result in different heart problems and can reduce the quality of life of someone.

Fiber is great in many ways; it also helps in weight loss and reduces the risk of getting into depression and anxiety because of the decluttering power it possesses.

You should increase your intake of fibers to increase your general body wellness and mental health.

Chewing Gum and Vagus Nerve Stimulation

When battling indigestion, chewing gum can help to increase bowel movement, aiding digestion and relieving stress that comes with constipation.

Gum chewing helps to release a certain hormone into the body which helps to stimulate the vagus nerve. This stimulation of the vagus nerve results in smooth digestion and stress reduction.

Chewing gum may be seen as a stressful exercise because of how it stresses the tooth and also may cause tooth decay, and sometimes it may be a distraction for someone who wants to be focused, but it's a quick way of stimulating your hormone and getting out of anxiety and stress.

Chapter Four: Polyvagal Theory

It has been said earlier that the vagus nerve is the calming aspect of the nervous system, which reverses the action of the adrenaline that functions in alerting the body against danger and harmful events for flight or fight.

The nervous system has always been seen and discussed as two parts that are acting antagonistic to each other (sympathetic and parasympathetic), but the discovery of the polyvagal theory introduced the third aspect of the nervous system which seeks to talk about the interplay of activation and the calming part of the nervous system which is as a result of the influence of a nerve.

Stephen Porges was the one who discovered this polyvagal theory and makes it more interesting by calling it a social engagement system. Polyvagal theory comprises neuroscientific facts as well as psychological and evolutionary claims about the function of the vagus nerve in emotional regulation, its connection to social life, and its involvement in the responses to fear and agitations.

The polyvagal theory centrally focuses on the structure and the functions of the efferent branches of the vagus nerve, which originates from the brain, specifically from the medulla oblongata.

The polyvagal theory seeks to bring balance between the mobilization and immobilization stage by introducing the social engagement and connection where a patient learns to interpret certain facial expressions and vocalizations to determine whether to run, defend himself or herself, or relax and calm down.

Understanding polyvagal theory is very essential for the well-being of a traumatized patient to avoid living a life of unnecessary anxiety and depression.

The Three Stages of Response

Stephen Porges explained the three stages that are involved in the growth of the autonomic nervous system of human beings. Instead of him just telling us about the system of balance the theory offers between the parasympathetic and sympathetic nervous system. Stephen described the stages involved in the autonomic nervous system development.

These three stages involved are listed below.

Immobilization

This is the oldest of them all, and it takes part in the immobilization responses. The back or the dorsal aspect of the vagus nerve responds to different dangers and frightening situations which make us swing into action or become immobile. When we are faced with scary situations, we can become so petrified and even freeze. As a result of the frightening situation, immobilization can happen instead of flight or slowing down

The immobilization stage is a very demanding and stressful one for trauma patients, and some remain in this stage of being vegatative for a very long time. Most times it is as a result of the brain shutting down at the point of the incidence.

When the fight or flight responses are too high for the victim, it may be too shocking and as a result, you may freeze. At this stage, the patient or victim needs every help they can find to remain alive and regain their control.

Mobilization

This is the sympathetic stage of our body system. It is the stage that sets us in motion when we are faced with danger and scary situations; we swing immediately into action as a result of the release of the adrenaline in the body to fight off the adversary or the enemy or run away to avoid the danger. The polyvagal theory suggests that the mobilization stage is the next phase to be devolved in the evolutionary system.

The mobilization stage requires a lot of work, and it is mostly the most developed of the three stages. If the victim can recover from immobilization and develop the mobilization stage, then he or she can connect with others for maximum social engagement.

It is the stage when the patient learns to step out, communicate, relearn certain things, and regain their mind for proper functioning. This is very essential and important for healthy living in society.

Social Engagement

Social engagement is the new stage added to the hierarchy. Its source is found in the front side of the vagus nerve, and it is this part that responds to the feelings of security and connection. This social engagement helps to feel secure and calm.

As we move and interact with our world, there are often moments when we feel secure or even feel nervous because of the dangers around us or feel discomfort. The polyvagal theory suggests the fact that this world is fluid for everyone, and we have the power to move in and out of these various places within these stages of responses.

As we go through life engaging with the world, there are inevitably those moments when we will feel safe and others in which we will feel discomfort or danger. Polyvagal theory suggests that this space is fluid for us and we can move in and out of these different places within the hierarchy of responses.

While away from home you may receive calls about armed robbery burgling your house and freeze and still experience anxiety during the journey. Your ability to maneuver fluidly between the experiences is polyvagal theory in action.

When we understand this theory then we will know its level of practicality in our day-to-day life. Polyvagal theory applies to our everyday life; we always have reasons to participate in social engagements, we have experienced overwhelming situations at the same time and still faced with situations that demand our immediate mobilization.

Stephen Porges was truly a deep thinker who analyzed our day-to-day lives to coin out this theory as it applies to our lives.

Sometimes trying situations can get us trapped, and we feel helpless and unable to move out of the situation. At this stage, your body increasingly feels danger and anxiety moves you into a deeper stage of immobilization; You can get trapped and frozen, numb as a result of the dorsal vagus nerve that's been influenced by this incidence.

When this happens, you enter a state of dissociation from the environment. An example can be a verbal or sexual abuse that leaves many dumbed and surprised.

Polyvagal Theory and its Impact on Traumatic Situations

Most times traumatized patients are left immobilized due to the level of pain that followed the experience or events, and as such, they become hypersensitive and can easily think they sense or scan any danger that wants to come around next time.

This is the issue with patients who have had to deal with traumatic experiences before is that they become paranoid and suspicious without any reason; their ability to actually detect danger is impaired. Although, our aim is to ensure you experience healing from these traumatic experiences by engaging your vagus nerve but understanding how to navigate through these difficult situations ensures it never happens again.

Understanding this polyvagal theory will help us understand how to interact more fluidly with other people around us in order to feel safe and secure. When the importance of stimulation of the vagus nerve is understood, then a traumatic patient can move from immobility to mobility and pick up signals when there is danger, which swing them into action to run for their dear lives or defend themselves by attacking back.

This theory makes us understand when we are safe and relaxed and when we are in danger and need to flee in combination with the adrenaline that is released into the body for action. When we are safe and secure the vagusstoff substance is released into the body to make us feel relaxed and calmed.

Sometimes, stressful situations will make a trauma patient remember the past traumatic experience they had. Maybe the light, someone's voice, a color, sound, or familiar face reminded them of past trauma, and they can prepare them to run for their lives or sound an alarm with that trigger.

An example of a traumatic experience is rape.

Rape can be very traumatizing that the victim may remain frozen or even shut down unexpectedly as a result of the shock that comes from the experience. Such a person may remain in an immobile state of mind for a while, disturbed by different dreams of the event and may lose connection with people around them.

If this person sees a similar color of cloth of the rapist, or hears a similar voice, sees something that looks familiar, they may be scared and keep entering the immobile state till they are helped out and reconnected socially.

For a traumatic patient, fight or flight may not be registered as an option in their body due to an experience that has affected their vagus nerve, but with polyvagal theory, over time they can learn to interact and experience natural healing as a result of the stimulation of the vagus nerve.

Polyvagal Theory and Human Connection with Others

The vagus nerve has extensive branches into the body distributed to different parts of the body but originated from the brain step specifically the medulla oblongata. This vagus nerve can impact our social connection and engagement by modulating our facial expression and also our vocalization.

As a result of these facial expressions and the intonation (vocalization), humans can scan for dangers around in our interactions with others. We are designed to connect with others and we cant see the signs of connection, and by doing this, we begin to watch out for ourselves.

Humans can sense or discern trust in people, and this discernment will determine our level of safety and comfort with others, but if our discernment or gut feelings are not right, then we begin to think of the next step of action for flight or fight.

As we begin to grow in trust for ourselves and feel safe around ourselves, we begin to interact and grow in vulnerabilities with each other and even bond. This is one of the most important aspects of the polyvagal theory.

These facial expressions and vocalization have been important tools mostly used by the legal workers in detecting armed individuals or individuals with bad intentions. When we learn to pay attention to these things we will grow our sensitivity and ability to detect danger from afar and either stay away or move closer.

Sometimes, we wonder how some people can pick up certain communications through facial expressions or pick up on expressions of love through just the sound of a voice. It is this theory that can explain it.

The polyvagal theory seeks to explain attachment with people, non-verbal (facial) communications and emotional regulations.

Polyvagal Theory and Client's Assistant

When we are in contact with someone having mental health issues or traumatized patients, what is expected of us is to observe their social behaviors and interactions recognize what is actually happening for them to be reacting this way; then you show them love and help them get accustomed to the environment to feel safe and secure. You can help them get adjusted to people's facial expressions, appearances, and normal interactions among people in that environment that may seem strange to them.

Sometimes these patients may grow to be scared of every and anything around them because of their vegetative state over time which made them dumb for a while. You have that responsibility of making them understand the need for interpersonal relationships, interactions with others, and how to play safely. Although this may take a while for them to adjust, it will be helpful to give them necessary support.

There was a case of a woman who was happily married to her husband and kids with a very loving family. One day, she was rushing out with her car when she had a ghastly motor accident, and she remained in this vegetative state for a very long time because the accident was too sudden and she was traumatized and remained numb to the world.

A few years later, she opened her eyes and couldn't even recognize anyone. She suffered memory loss and couldn't remember her name, or even her address, so she remained at the hospital. A few years later, the policeman who found her on the road when she had the accident and had been taking care of her till she recovered took her in and fell in love with her.

Deep down, she knew she had a past and was a happy one but she couldn't remember what her past was all about. Anytime they stepped out together, the traffic signs and even the road would look familiar and the pains she feels, the anxiety each time she sees these familiar things are disturbing.

Then her new husband began to teach her how to deal with these anxieties, worries, and fear of the unknown and calm down. He began to teach her how to feel safe and secure in the environment and trust people for who they are. This went on for months until she accepted her new life and moved on from her unknown past. This was until she met her real husband, who showed her pictures that got her mobilized after reflections.

This is the best we can do to help our loved ones who battle with these same traumatic incidents, they will need to feel safe, secure and get to trust everyone around them and stay calm instead of the paranoia reactions and the flight and fight response at every slight signal they feel whether harmful or helpful.

In our social environment, we are faced with different things daily that should impact our nervous system to different degrees; they produce anxiety and worry in us. From political news to bad news from a loved one, if care is not taken, then we get our minds adjusted to these everyday troublesome news stories and incidences, and at every slight signal, our next line of action is flight. We must balance our responses to our environment and learn to interact with everyone by differentiating voices and facial expressions, connecting, and networking effectively for balance.

From these explanations of polyvagal theory and its applications to our social interactions, connections and dissociations, we can see that the autonomic nervous system forms the basis of our life experiences. It is upon us that our lives find expressions, and our ability to move between different stages of this theory, will determine our efficiency and effectiveness in society.

From a polyvagal perspective, the autonomic nervous system is the foundation upon which all lived experience exists. It explains how we move through engaging with the world (of activity and of interactions with people) through connecting, disconnecting, and attuning.

Understanding the application of polyvagal theory in our lives will help us in giving maximum attention to someone and help them recover from any traumatic experiences; we can help them experience natural healing and get them to pick up signals, recognize danger signals, and respond to these signals to prevent them from experiencing trauma all over again.

Conclusion

The vagus nerve is one of the most crucial nerves in the human body, and its natural healing power has been greatly ignored by many today. The vagus nerve is the tenth cranial nerve of the cranial nerves in the body, and the longest nerve as well. It is called the vagus nerve because it has extensive branches around the body, and as such, it is a wandering nerve.

Our general wellness is determined by the health of this nerve because of its significance and the certain functions it performs in the body. Understanding the anatomy of this nerve, its functions, and branches in the body will give us an understanding of how to leverage its features in order to heal, live with a better mood, be almost free of unnecessary stress and anxiety, and most importantly, have a quality life.

Trauma, anxiety, depression, hoarseness of voice, speech impairment, and others are symptoms of dysfunctional vagus nerve in the body, and if left untreated, may result in certain diseases in the body like obesity, arthritis, cardiac arrest, high blood pressure, inflammatory diseases, and other issues that may reduce the quality of the life of a man.

The vagus nerve also helps us to live a healthy social life. When we begin to understand that the vagus nerve affects our moods and our vocalization, and these determine how we connect with other people and have a good social life, then we will understand how important it is that we keep our vagus nerve stimulated always.

There are certain things many people do casually without knowing how these things influence their lives; they just do them to derive pleasure and enjoy the moment, but if we understand the effects of these activities, then we will be intentional about these activities.

There are different ways by which we can stimulate our vagus nerve naturally to tap into the healing power of this nerve. All these exercises have been established scientifically, and there have been countless testimonies of how vagus nerve stimulation has helped cure depression, anxiety, arthritis, and trauma.

Activities that help stimulate your vagus nerve include: deep breathing exercises, chewing gum, sleeping on the right side of the body, increasing the intake of fibers, singing, humming, chanting, meditation on beautiful and inspiring quotes, meditation on gratitude and kindness of God, having healthy social connections. Doing these helps you to relieve stress, halt feelings of depression or anxiety, and most importantly, improve the quality of your health.

The vagus nerve helps reverse the work of the sympathetic nerve in the body. Sympathetic nerves are involved in the fight or flight response to scary and frightening events or situations; during these events, adrenaline is released into the body which alerts us and gets us ready for the next action of defense.

During this event, the blood pressure of the body increases as a result of the release of adrenaline into the body, this leads to an increase in the cardiac output, anxiety setting in, then you either fight or take flight.

The vagus nerve acts by releasing a substance called vagusstoff into the body which brings about a calming effect. This calming effect helps to reduce the blood pressure, cardiac output, and brings you out of the depressive mood into a relaxed mood.

Stress also can lead to the release of adrenaline in the body which may result in depression, anxiety, blood pressure increment, and other things related. We all have our stressors and understanding our stressors will help us know how to handle them. When stress is prolonged in the body, it reduces the quality of life of someone.

No human can function at his or her best when stressed because of the mental instability stress brings. When you make these vagus nerve stimulation exercises as part of your routines or add them to your to-do list, then you will always stay stress-free with the strong mind needed to hit your goals.

If the vagus nerve fails to stimulate at this stage, the blood pressure remains high, the cardiac output will remain high, and the mood will remain depressed as you remain anxious. This can result in cardiac arrest and other heart problems that can reduce the quality of life of an individual.

This is why we must by all means avoid vagus nerve dysfunctionality. The vagus nerve truly plays major roles in the body. The excessive stimulation of the nerve also has effects on the emotions and may result in certain kinds of diseases in the body, and as such, it must be kept regulated.

When the vagus nerve is too stimulated, the heartbeat slows down and this leads to a shortage of oxygen in the brain as a result of the low pumping of the blood into the brain that carries oxygen. This will lead to memory loss, chronic pains, arrhythmias, and other diseases.

The polyvagal theory seeks to bring balance to the two parts of the nervous system; the sympathetic and parasympathetic system by introducing social engagement and connections. It helps us to understand the connection between the brain, the heart, and the internal organs receiving information from the vagus nerve.

Polyvagal theory speaks about the three levels of development of the nervous system. These include: immobilization, mobilization, and social engagement and connection. A traumatic patient can be left in a vegetative state for long as a result of the freezing, shock, and shut down and become immobile.

When they recover, they lose their ability to pick up signals and respond effectively to fight/flight mode, becoming uncomfortable with every and anything, losing trust in people around them, and losing the ability to feel safe and secure.

When we get this knowledge of polyvagal theory, we can help get the traumatized patients to get comfortable in such an atmosphere by teaching them how to discern and sense signals, how to respond to different signals (either to relax when there is no danger or run when faced with dangers), how to recognize faces and tell if someone is dangerous, and how to recognize different tone voices that give off different signals.

These are very important for these traumatic patients to know for a good social connection, meaning they must understand different vocalizations and facial expressions to get them out of their immobile states to mobile and to social engagement.

The vagus nerve can get dysfunctional through brain injury, surgery involving internal organs, and other traumas. It is important we understand these revelations about the vagus nerve for us to know how to improve our lives because it is the sole nerve responsible for the quality of life in regards to the general mental and physical wellness of the body.

Our mental well-being is essential for our productivity, and the vagus nerve provides us with strong mental wellness and helps keep our sanity.

If you enjoyed this book in anyway, an honest review is always appreciated!

www.ingramcontent.com/pod-product-compliance
Lightning Source LLC
Chambersburg PA
CBHW030917080526
44589CB00010B/350